American Life League's
Life Guide Series
Volume 2

The Facts
About
Birth Control

American Life League's
Life Guide Series

Volume 2

The Facts About Birth Control

Judie Brown

American Life League, Inc.
Stafford, Virginia

ISBN 1-890712-13-2

American Life League,Inc.
P.O. Box 1350
Stafford, VA 22555

Acknowledgements

This booklet would not have been possible without the assistance and kind suggestions of Sheena Talbot, Rebecca Lindstedt, Kate Fitzgerald, and John Cavanaugh-O'Keefe.

Dedication

To all those who have been deceived by the birth control movement and victimized by the sexual revolutionaries of our day.

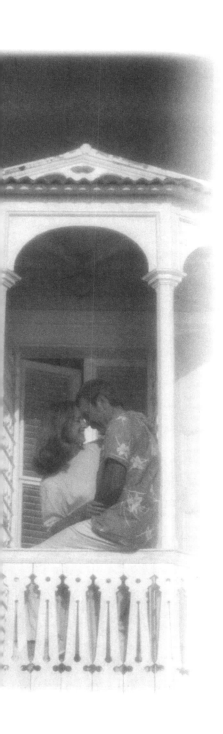

Table of Contents

Table of Contents

- What is the history of birth control?

- How do we describe birth control?
  — Family Planning
  — Contraception
  — Birth Control

- Does this mean that artificial methods are the problem, rather than the label we use?

- Why is it a problem if I don't intend to have a baby?
  — Viewpoint #1—I want to have sex outside of marriage

  Figure 1:Gonorrhea Cases, Females Aged 15–19

  — Viewpoint #2—I want protection
  — Viewpoint #3—I want freedom
  — Viewpoint #3—I want a risk-free relationship

- What do the experts say?

- What are the most popular forms of birth control?
  — Diaphragm and Spermicide
  — Condom

- What are the birth control methods that cause early abortion?

  Figure 2: The Human Embryo—from fertilization until the fifth week after conception

  — Birth control pill (oral contraceptive)
  — IUD
  — Norplant
  — DepoProvera
  — Morning-after pill (emergency contraception)

- Why is it such a big secret that these chemicals and devices kill?

- Who is telling the truth?

- Some pregnancies are unplanned or unwanted—or both! What about that?

  — Birth control and facing the baby
  — Medical abortion as birth control

- Why do some people call these drugs birth control and not just call them abortion drugs?

  — MTX (Methotrexate) + Misoprostol
  — RU-486 + Misoprostol

- What are the long-term implications for our society of the latest advances in the birth control/abortion field?

- Is there any good news about birth control?

- So married couples should rethink their use of birth control too?

- One final thought

Introduction

Since the early 1960's, when birth control came into vogue, there has been an emphasis on "protecting" men and women from having children. There has been little attention paid to the reasons why birth control works or how it might affect a person's attitudes toward sex, marriage or family. It is the purpose of this book to address these aspects of birth control.

I hope to clarify some basic things people should know and understand before making the decision to use birth control. For those who have already decided to use birth control, I invite you to give it a second look.

This book is designed to help you through the maze by answering your many questions about birth control. Human beings can make informed choices in their lives only if they have all the facts.

I will offer brief descriptions of various forms of birth control—how they are supposed to work, why they don't work, and what the dangers are. You will also learn the reasons why the so-called sexual revolution of the 1960's has not fulfilled the promises of fewer abortions and happier lives. Contrary to popular opinion, abortions have increased because of the acceptance of birth control.

Judie Brown, President
American Life League, Inc.

Birth Control: The Record

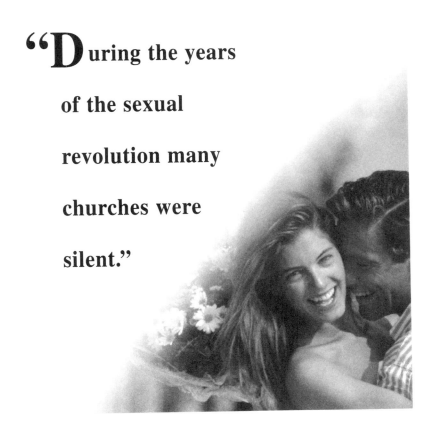

"During the years

of the sexual

revolution many

churches were

silent."

Birth Control: The Record

What is the history of birth control?

Throughout history, people have attempted to control their fertility in one way or another. Before 1930, however, such efforts were sporadic. People who promoted the idea of "using something" foreign to the body were looked upon with skepticism. Laws prohibited, for example, the sale and distribution of such products. Health and public policy leaders condemned birth control as a threat to the family. In fact, as late as 1915, when Margaret Sanger (the founder of Planned Parenthood) and others attempted to promote artificial intervention to "end pregnancy" or "bring on a woman's period," they were described as fanatics. Sanger spent time in jail because she was promoting illicit behavior and illegal material. Before 1930, no large body of opinion makers—and no church anywhere in the world—supported artificial birth control.

In 1930, the tide began to change. In England, the Anglican Church held the Lambeth Conference, at which it debated whether married couples could use artificial methods of birth control—on rare occasions, and for serious reasons. Under these narrow circumstances, the Anglican Church accepted birth control as a licit practice. This one church's determination had negative results no one could have predicted. The decision was a break in the history of Christianity, which had always presented a united front in opposition to any activity or practice that would deny the natural law by giving man dominion over God's design for procreation.

After that time, groups promoting the birth control ideology slowly gained strength in developed countries. In 1961, a Planned Parenthood group in Connecticut decided to challenge the state law that forbade the provision of artificial methods of birth control to married couples. Planned Parenthood's position was that couples, whether married or unmarried, should be free to choose the manner in which they planned their children. In 1965, the U.S. Supreme Court (in *Griswold* v. *Connecticut*) ruled that the state law was invalid. Its decision struck down similar state laws across the nation. Proponents of artificial methods of birth control attained a level of respectability that led to Congressional hearings, advertising in favor of birth control and, ultimately, the decision of the U.S. government to fund programs that focused on artificial birth control.

This is not an accident of history. The birth control pill was gaining notoriety in the early 1960's. The idea of both married couples and singles having access to artificial methods of birth control and abortion was gaining public acceptance. Backers of population control among the poor in our nation and around the world pushed for government programs that would foster their ideology. These powerful groups wanted to see fewer numbers of the poor and minority races, and they were staunch advocates of birth control and abortion.

During the 1960's, sexual values were changing, attitudes toward the permanency of marriage were faltering and social planners were seeking new and better ways for people who engaged in sexual relations (whether married or single) to effectively avoid pregnancy.

During these years of the "sexual revolution" many churches were silent. The U.S. government was under increasing pressure not only to approve the practice of birth control but also to take an active part in its advocacy. The pressure succeeded. In 1970, the federal government authorized and funded the first government birth control program. Shortly thereafter, in 1973, the Supreme Court struck down all laws prohibiting abortion. It was clear that the proponents of birth control had won the cultural argument. No longer would people have to worry about the moral implications of acting against nature, because the government was in charge of the question.

In the late 1960's, morality in matters of sexual practice became a question of law rather than a question of truth. The results have been devastating.

Over the last 30 years, for example, the number of known venereal diseases has grown from 5 to 50. The divorce rate has skyrocketed. The number of out-of-wedlock pregnancies has risen, and in America alone there are more than one million surgical abortions each year. In addition, millions of unseen abortions occur because of the ways in which certain types of birth control actually work.

Abortion and birth control are now key components of the U.S. government's population programs in Third World nations. Poor people in other countries would like to learn how to improve the lives of their family members, but the United States offers only one answer—smaller families. This is called eugenics. It is at the foundation of American public policy, a policy based on the philosophy of Margaret Sanger and her followers, who fought poverty by offering birth control as the only viable solution.

Before 1930, no church, no political system, and no culture had ever adopted birth control as an acceptable way of relating to members of the opposite sex. After 1930, as history has shown, decay began to erode the public morality and the personal moral attitudes of millions.

How do we describe birth control?

For the purposes of this book, *birth control* means artificial (unnatural) devices or chemicals. There is an important difference between natural and artificial methods of spacing children. Artificial (unnatural) birth control includes the Pill, the intrauterine device (IUD), the condom, the diaphragm, spermicides, Norplant, DepoProvera and other unnatural means of "avoiding" pregnancy.

You frequently hear references to either *family planning* or *contraception* or *birth control*. Today all three names usually refer to one simple idea: taking an action (using birth control) to avoid the natural consequences of another action (sexual relations).

Let's see what these specific words mean in simple terms.

Family planning

This sounds like two people are married and they are preparing to have a family. They want to proceed with some kind of plan so that they either do not have too many children, or so that the children they do have are spaced according to the parents' will and desire. If this is what comes to mind, then those involved in the propaganda battle favoring artificial methods of birth control have won the word game.

In today's culture, *family planning* is equated with an unmarried person seeking a method of *protection* from pregnancy or disease so this person can have *sex outside of marriage*. Indeed, statistics show that many people do engage in sexual relations outside of marriage. Throughout our culture, there are messages suggesting that such relations are acceptable and perfectly healthy.

There are places, such as family planning clinics, school-based clinics or health clinics, where a person can get the artificial *family planning* method he or she is seeking. Some of these methods—condoms and spermicides—are available at grocery stores and other retail outlets because no physician's prescription is required.

Family planning represents a collection of unnatural substances and devices designed to encourage sex without consequences, sex outside of marriage, sex for the sake of sex. Though the phrase *family planning* should refer to the idea of planning a family, it has been redefined by proponents of birth control and abortion.

Contraception

If you look this word up in the dictionary, you will see that it literally means *against conception*. This definition implies that if a contraceptive is used, no pregnancy will occur. According to the dictionary, contraception is supposed to *prevent* or *protect*. In this sense, a contraceptive is designed to *prevent* pregnancy or disease, or to *protect* you from getting pregnant or contracting a sexually transmitted disease (STD) such as gonorrhea or HIV. True contraceptives never cause abortions. The only true contraceptives are condoms, diaphragms and spermicides. But this does not necessarily mean they are safe, or that they will protect anyone from STD's.

Birth control

Birth control is an action taken to control the onset of pregnancy—or to control the outcome, if pregnancy does occur, by ending the pregnancy before the baby is born. This is the most truthful of the three terms we are discussing (family planning, contraception and birth control).

A person uses a type of unnatural birth control only if he or she is interested in avoiding a baby or a disease. Why would a healthy human being swallow a chemical or use a device for absolutely no reason? We can conclude that the person who uses an artificial form of birth control is doing so to avoid what he or she sees as a negative outcome—an undesirable result, a problem. However, chastity works far better in the long run.

Although some forms of birth control, such as condoms and spermicides, do not actually cause abortion, many other methods do. Remember the definition:

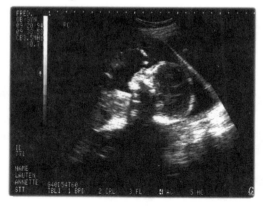

Birth control: An action taken to control the onset of pregnancy—or to control the outcome, if pregnancy does occur, *by ending the pregnancy before the baby is born.*

The Pill, the IUD and other methods act not only against pregnancy but also against the newly-conceived baby.

Does this means that artificial *methods* are the problem, rather than the label we use?

Yes. When the intent of the user is negative, the result also is negative. If the user is saying no—no to self-control, no to a possible baby, no to accepting the results of sexual intercourse—then he or she may easily decide to surgically abort the child if the method fails. In fact, the people who promote birth control in our society are often quoted as saying that surgical abortion is—and *must* be—a backup to *failed* birth control!

It is the negative intent of the birth control user that causes the moral problem.

Why is it a problem if I don't intend to have a baby?

If you have sexual relations and still don't want a baby, that's self-serving and an abuse of freedom.

Let's examine the various viewpoints of people who use birth control and see what we can learn.

Figure 1: Gonorrhea Cases, Females aged 15-19

By the Thousands

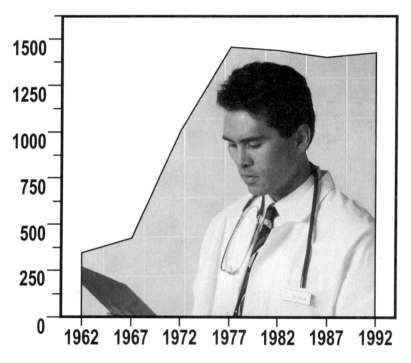

Source: U.S. Department of Health and Human Services,
Public Health Service

VIEWPOINT #1: I want to have sex outside of marriage.

This viewpoint is very popular today, yet thousands of unmarried women are getting pregnant, and thousands of men and women are suffering from STD's, including HIV/AIDS. Look at Figure #1. This viewpoint brings these results.

VIEWPOINT #2: I want protection.

What else could this mean except protection *from* something—a baby or a disease? This is really a false sense of security. Although a person may think that a particular form of birth control will protect him or her from pregnancy or disease, the facts do not support this. In far too many cases, children are conceived and then destroyed by the birth control method in use; and, as the statistics show, STD's occur with greater frequency because of promiscuity.

In addition, the negative outlook of the birth control user does not help a relationship. Sex itself takes over as the primary focus of a friendship that should be based on respect, trust, mutual commitment and love. Loving someone doesn't just happen as an isolated incident or because of a single moment in time. A love that grows is a love that accepts the other human being as someone deserving of respect, patience and a potential lifetime commitment—not a one-night stand.

Maybe the birth control user really wants protection from making a pledge of one's total being—a commitment that will grow. Maybe he or she wants protection from love, too.

VIEWPOINT #3: I want freedom.

In the context of using birth control, this means independence from any long-term relationship with another human being. It means that the individual does not want the responsibility for his actions and would prefer to be "free" of the consequences.

VIEWPOINT #4: I want a risk-free relationship.

This means that a man or woman is willing to take a risk, but does not want to be burdened with the outcome. These people believe that birth control will provide a shield between them and anything they might wish to avoid.

Professionals who study human relationships, including about current cultural attitudes regarding sexual relations, say these attitudes are real. They cause heartache, and sometimes—if things don't work out—they can cause serious illness and death.

What do the experts say?

Dr. Hugh K. Barber wrote in an editorial in the first issue of *The Female Patient* in 1976:

> With the introduction of oral contraceptives (birth control pills) in 1956, a new era arrived with a tremendous impact on medicine, religion, philosophy, sociology and even geopolitical thinking. Many women have been moving from the kitchen and the home to competitive life in the outside world.[1]

I am not suggesting there is something wrong with women who choose to work outside the home. Many must do this. Others want to pursue a career and raise a family. But it is troubling that Dr. Barber failed to note that many men can now travel an easier road with women if they don't want to pursue engagement and marriage. Birth control provides men with a kind of hold-harmless agreement.

Lionel Tiger, an evolutionary anthropologist, wrote in *U.S. News and World Report* in 1996:

I think the introduction of widespread contraceptive use in the 1960's caused this revolutionary breakdown between men and women. It put biological disputes at the center of our national life—women's rights, abortion, out-of-wedlock births . . . the pill emancipated women and placed into question existing moral and religious systems that focused on controlling sexual behavior.[2]

Dr. Janet Smith, who teaches philosophy at the University of Dallas, said:

Far from being a check to the sexual revolution, contraception is the fuel that facilitated the beginning of the sexual revolution and enables it to continue to rage. In the past, many men and women refrained from illicit sexual unions simply because they were not prepared for the responsibilities of parenthood. But once a fairly reliable contraceptive appeared on the scene, the barrier to sex outside the confines of marriage fell. The connection between sex and love also fell quickly.[3]

The basic problem with the practice of birth control and its wide acceptance in the culture is moral breakdown—the practice of sexual unions that are wrong. We see disrespect of the marriage covenant—the promise of lifelong love for one another—something that once was the norm in society. The mechanical aspects of the sexual act between a man and a woman have become goals in and of themselves without regard to moral implications. As the culture has increasingly accepted birth control, we have also seen an acceptance of sex outside of marriage (promiscuity), sex with people other than one's spouse (infidelity), and divorce.

This is one of the reasons that there are so many children today in single-parent homes. With the advent of birth control practice came an acceptance of sexual relations as distinctly separate from marriage. The two people who engage in a sexual relationship no longer feel compelled to accept a lifelong commitment or the children who come into being as a result of their sexual activity.

Because birth control fails, human beings do conceive other human beings. But no one in a relationship based on sexual freedom is prepared to accept the responsibility for the children created. Morally this is wrong, but culturally it is the norm.

These are some pretty tough comments. And even though nobody ever has all the answers, it may be time to take a closer look at birth control—not only for reasons of health but also for reasons of truth. Clearly there is reason to believe that birth control is not such a good idea.

Birth Control:
The Mechanics

"A perfectly healthy woman

takes potentially harmful

foreign material into

her body."

Birth Control: The Mechanics

What are the most popular forms of birth control?

The birth control methods most common today include the diaphragm, spermicides, the condom, the Pill, the IUD, Norplant, DepoProvera, the morning-after pill, medical abortions (methotrexate plus miso-prostol, and RU-486 plus misoprostol) and surgical abortion, which is touted as necessary when other forms of contraception fail.

Each of these methods has different properties, and they are alleged to accomplish certain things if used properly. Below is a list of the different types of birth control, a brief description of each, and the problems associated with each.

The facts should become clear to you as you review this material. Please note that everything is footnoted. There are plenty of references you can seek out and examine yourself.

Diaphragm and Spermicide

A diaphragm is a small, flexible device made of rubber or plastic that fits over the cervix (the lower, narrow part of the uterus). It is usually inserted just prior to sexual intercourse.

Diaphragms vary according to size. The first time a woman decides to use this method, she must be fitted for a diaphragm. If she continues to rely on the diaphragm, she may need to be fitted again after a period of time.

Most women use the diaphragm with a spermicide, which is a gel-like substance that is designed to kill sperm.

Problems:

Urinary tract infections are common among sexually active young women. The risk is strongly associated with recent sexual intercourse, recent use of a diaphragm with spermicide, and a history of recurrent urinary tract infections.[4]

The urinary tract infection (or acute cystitis) occurs about seven million times a year. These infections occur most frequently in women 18–22 years of age. The first signs are itching and a burning sensation during urination. Treatment is available, but the infection is painful and can recur often.

Condom

This latex contraceptive was originally designed for use by men, but recently a female condom has been introduced to the market with limited success. The purpose of the condom is to stop the sperm from reaching the woman's cervix. If the sperm are unable to enter the cervix, pregnancy will not occur.

Problems:

Sperm and the AIDS Virus

While a condom may stop sperm, tiny holes in the latex may allow HIV, the virus that causes AIDS, to pass through. Thus, "safe sex" is not as safe as condom proponents would have you believe. An article in the February 1992 issue of *Applied and Environmental Microbiology* reported that the HIV-1 virus is only four millionths of an inch in diameter. It is *three times smaller* than the herpes virus, *60 times smaller* than the syphilis spirochete, and *50 to 450 times smaller than sperm.*[5]

Condom + Spermicide

Some people advocate the use of spermicide containing nonoxynol-9 to prevent HIV infection. However, researchers have not been able to prove whether this spermicide actually protects against other types of STD's.[6,7]

What are the birth control methods that cause early abortion?

Birth control pills, IUD's and the new chemical birth control methods (Norplant, DepoProvera, methotrexate + misoprostol, RU-486) are quite different from the barrier methods and spermicides. In each case, the woman must either swallow pills, have a device inserted into her womb or her arm, or have a chemical injected into her body. In each of these cases, a perfectly healthy woman is taking potentially harmful foreign material into her body—not because she is treating a problem such as a headache, but because she is hoping to avoid pregnancy.

The Alan Guttmacher Institute (the research arm of Planned Parenthood) reports that "half of all abortion patients in 1987 were practicing contraception [including the Pill] during the month in which they conceived."[8]

Even today, there is a great deal of long-term health information that is not known, or at least not reported, about these various methods.

For example, these birth control methods at least occasionally (or in some cases, always) work to cause early abortion in the woman's body. Each method can allow pregnancy to begin and then, because of the manner in which it functions in the woman's body, act to kill the newly conceived little boy or girl. The vast majority of women who use these various methods may not even realize that these early abortions are happening.

Let's take a moment to study the development of the human being in his mother's womb, especially during the first few days. Please see Figure #2, and read the descriptions carefully.

A. Ovulation. The ovum (egg), which is surrounded by a protective covering, is released into the Fallopian tube.[9]

B. Fertilization. A person begins the first day of his or her life within the mother's body. At this point the 23 chromosomes carried by the sperm and the 23 chromosomes carried by the egg combine to form a new one-cell human being, or human embryo, containing 46 chromosomes. The new person is called a human zygote.[10] Each of the 46 chromosomes is composed of genes, or units of DNA, that contain all of the genetic information of the new person.[11] No genetic information is either gained or lost.[12] The zygote is already genetically an individual[13] human being and a "he" or a "she."[14]

C. 24 hours. The zygote divides to form a two-cell embryo.[15]

Figure 2: The Human Embryo—from fertilization until the fifth week after conception

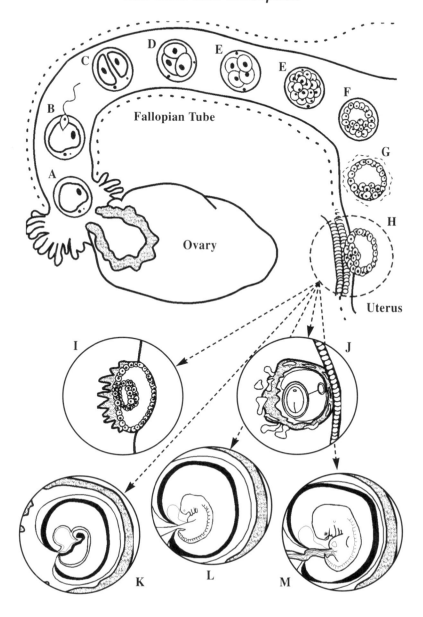

D. Second day. One of the cells divides. Now the embryo has three cells.[15]

E. Third day. The embryo consists of four cells which divide to make eight, then 16 cells. The 16-cell stage is called the morula stage.[15]

F. Fourth day. Early blastocyst stage. The embryo has entered the uterus.[16]

G. Fifth day. Late blastocyst stage. The outer protective membrane begins to disintegrate as implantation approaches.[17]

H. Implantation of the embryo into the wall of the uterus begins between the sixth and seventh day.[17]

I. Eighth day. Implantation continues.[17]

J. Embryo implantation is complete about day 14. On day 15, the primitive streak (migration of key cells toward the center of the embryo) begins to appear.[17]

K. Third week. The heart begins to beat; neural folds and the major divisions of the brain appear, as well as somites (the neural crest and the beginnings of the internal ear and the eye).[18]

L. Fourth week. The primitive streak begins to disappear. About 30 pairs of somites are present; a large, distinct head and limb buds begin to appear; major outlines of brain and eye vesicles are observable, along with the beginnings of the central nervous system, notochord, mouth and pharynx, body cavity and the basis of the skeleton.[19]

M. Fifth week. The face is taking shape; the forehead, eyes, nostrils and mouth are evident; external ears are beginning; hand and foot plates appear in the limb buds.[20]

Because it is a scientific fact that the life of every human being begins at fertilization, we have to wonder why the manufacturers of birth control chemicals and devices don't simply tell women all the facts. For example, some Pill package inserts will state that the method works to prevent "nidation." This means that the implantation of the tiny boy or girl in the womb of the mother is prevented and the human being dies. But most women who read such a word would not realize that it means "prevents the continued life of the tiny human being."

The Birth Control Pill (Oral Contraceptive)

There are many different brands and combinations of these pills, and many different companies producing them. There are some general statements we can make about all of them, though, relying on pharmacists who have studied these chemicals and know how they work.

Oral contraceptives work in three different ways. They:

- prevent ovulation (release of an egg from the ovary);

- cause changes in the cervical mucus, which block or slow the travel of the sperm; and

- prevent implantation of the newly conceived baby into the lining of the mother's womb, thus causing an abortion.

Oral contraceptives send a chemical message to the rest of the body, giving it the impression the oral contraceptive user is constantly pregnant 12 months of the year.

All vital organs of the woman are affected by the powerful steroids in oral contraceptives.

Problems:

If the oral contraceptive user takes antibiotics or anti-convulsant prescription drugs while she is using the Pill, the chances of the Pill actually aborting a baby increase. Because there can be a drug interaction between the contraceptive pill and the second prescription drug, the Pill could become less reliable. Ovulation could occur any way, and the conception of a baby could take place.[22]

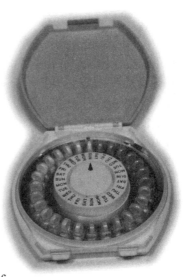

There is increasing research suggesting that oral contraceptives suppress the immune system. If the immune system is suppressed, the likelihood of contracting STD's, including HIV, increases.[23]

Side effects of oral contraceptives are wide-ranging, depending on the user, and include increased incidence of HIV, pelvic inflammatory disease, infertility, blood clots, breast cancer, stroke, cervical cancer and ectopic pregnancy.

What do professionals say about the Pill?

When the Pill was first approved for use in the United States in 1966, The Food and Drug Administration (FDA) Advisory Committee on Obstetrics and Gynecology issued this statement: "The oral contraceptives present society with problems unique in the history of human therapeutics. Never will so many people have taken such potent drugs voluntarily over such a protracted period for an objective other than the control of disease."[24]

Thirty years later, physician Ellen Grant said, "Preferred ignorance has caused us to close our eyes to the enormous increase in ill health of young women since the pill was introduced."[25]

The IUD (Intrauterine Device)

IUD's are not as popular in the United States as they were in the 1970's and 80's, but it is worthwhile to know how they work.

IUD's abort babies by means of copper or the synthetic hormone (progesterone) they contain. This interferes with natural processes in the uterus, preventing implantation of the tiny boy or girl. The manufacturers, however, do not describe their products with much accuracy, and you may be led to believe that there is no abortion occurring.

Problems:

Common side effects of IUD's include pelvic inflammatory disease, ectopic pregnancy, temporary or permanent sterility, perforation of the uterus, and endometriosis (inflammation of the lining of the uterus).

An IUD manufacturer's claim:

Alza is a corporation that manufactures Progestasert, an IUD that is described as an "intrauterine progesterone contraceptive system." This means that the chemical contained in the IUD acts in the woman's system. In a letter to ALL, the manufacturer insisted that its IUD is NOT an abortifacient.

Enclosed with the letter, to prove a point, was a 1989 article that claimed that because the embryonic baby (tiny boy or girl) disappeared from the womb and left no "marker," no one could claim that the IUD aborts.[26]

That is not true, because the IUD works in such a way that the uterine lining is made hostile to the little boy or girl. Whether the baby leaves a "marker" makes no difference if one is going to be scientifically accurate. If the baby had been able to implant in the wall of his mother's uterus, his life would have continued. If he cannot implant, he dies—and that is abortion.

Maybe someday the pharmaceutical companies will admit their intentional deception and begin telling the truth.

Norplant

This is a set of six narrow, soft plastic capsules that are implanted in a woman's upper arm. Norplant is said to last up to five years. Although Wyeth-Ayerst, the manufacturer, continues to claim that

Norplant does not cause early abortion, numerous studies show that Norplant does indeed abort tiny boys and girls.

Warning:

Class action lawsuits, representing more than 50,000 women, have been filed against the manufacturer of Norplant because of devastating side effects, including blindness, excessive bleeding, acne, hair loss, weight gain and physical pain. The FDA has warned that Norplant may also be linked to stroke and high blood pressure.

Norplant and the justice system

Facts about how Norplant is being used are also disturbing. In recent years, judges have ordered women to use Norplant as a condition of parole or as punishment because they have been convicted of child abuse. In addition, one medical journal claimed (and there have been many such articles) that teenage girls must be conditioned to accept Norplant because "35% of adolescents who stated they were sexually active reported using no contraception at first intercourse."[27]

DepoProvera

This is a drug (medroxyprogesterone, or DMPA) that is given to women in the form of an injection. This drug was originally approved for treatment of endometrial cancer. It was not until October 29, 1992, that the FDA allowed the Upjohn company to use this drug as a contraceptive. But again, this chemical aborts tiny boys and girls.

For women who use this form of birth control, DepoProvera injections are given every three months.

Problems:

In his book *A Consumer's Guide to the Pill and Other Drugs*, pharmacist John Wilks reports serious problems with DepoProvera, including risk of breast cancer among women younger than 25, irregular bleeding, suppression of bone density, and possible links with cervical cancer.[28] Other side effects can include increased risk of blood clots in the legs, lungs, heart, brain, and other major organs, and ectopic pregnancy.[29]

Morning-After Pill (Emergency Contraception)

These two terms are designed to deceive. Women are told that if they take double doses of the Pill—accurately described as mega-doses—within 72 hours after they have had sex, there will be no chance of pregnancy. The recommended dose is two to four birth control pills within 72 hours, with a second dose of two pills 12 hours later.[30] However, we know from scientific studies that if the woman is fertile, the sperm can fertilize the egg within mere hours of intercourse. At that point a new human being's life has already begun.

If a woman who is already pregnant takes these high doses, that tiny boy or girl will die. A mega-dose of the birth control pill can act to destroy the human being (embryo) before he or she has a chance to implant in the mother's uterus (a process that takes about five or six days). If the child does survive these chemicals, there is a high probability that he or she will be born with serious birth defects.

Problems:

Side effects for the woman can include nausea, vomiting, breast tenderness, and evidence of ectopic pregnancy. In addition, the potential for blood clot formation is increased because of the extremely high doses of these artificial hormones.[31]

Politics:

In the case of the so-called morning-after pill, the FDA held hearings in June 1996 to determine whether this practice of mega-dosing should be approved. Despite the risks, approval was granted.

Organizations such as Planned Parenthood wanted to have the government's approval to give the pills in this manner. When a similar effort was tried in 1994, it failed. However, the practice had already been going on for some time. Ann Landers told her readers about it in 1987.[32] But the promoters of this so-called answer to *unprotected sex* desired wider public acceptance of it.

No pharmaceutical companies asked for government approval for fear of opposition from the pro-life movement and lawsuits from women who were damaged by side effects.

Certain "family planning" and pro-abortion organizations have a vested interest in doing away with tiny boys and girls under the guise of helping women avoid an "unplanned" or "unwanted" pregnancy.

They say *avoid*, but they mean *kill*.

Why is it such a big secret that these chemicals and devices kill?

Medical and pharmaceutical professionals have de-cided to redefine the beginning of a human being's life so that women will never know that their babies are dying. Pregnancy itself has been redefined to advance a pro-death agenda in America.

As figure 2 (Page 21) shows clearly, by the time the baby (embryo or embryonic human being) implants at age 5 or 6 days, life is well on its way.

Who's telling the truth?

Here's what one newspaper reported:

"The [Center for Reproductive Law and Policy] considers morning-after pills a form of contraception since they block the fertilized egg from implanting into the uterine wall. Implantation, not fertilization, marks the beginning of pregnancy by some in the health community."[21]

In other words, even though basic scientific facts clearly show that a baby's life begins at fertilization, the advocates of birth control have revised this definition.

This alone should cause fear and distrust in the heart of every woman. If a physician or health care professional can so easily redefine the beginning of human life, and participate in that deception, what else might be hidden from the unsuspecting patient?

Note: All of the clinical information in this book has been verified by Pharmacists for Life International (PFLI). For details on how to contact PFLI for further information, see the REFERENCES FOR FURTHER READING section at the back of this book.

Birth Control:
The Consequences

"**N**ot only is the child going
to die, but many mothers
will also die—or be
maimed for life."

Birth Control:
The Consequences

Some pregnancies are unplanned or unwanted—or both! What about that?

When people start describing the existence of a baby in his mother's womb with negative terms such as unplanned or unwanted, they're really suggesting that the person who is carrying this child did not want to become pregnant. But if she truly did not want to be pregnant, why did she get sexually involved with anyone until she was married and prepared to welcome children into the world?

On the other hand, if a woman is already expecting a child, she is a mother who deserves assistance, support, love and compassion. She is in a situation that may be causing her distress, so the attitude of those around her should be one of encouragement. She should not be pressured to exercise the "choice" to end her child's life. She is a mother with a child. The only negativity in this situation arises from the unwillingness of people around her to sacrifice so that she can continue carrying her child and raise him or her to the best of her ability. Love her. Don't reject her and don't reject her child.

Birth control and facing the baby

Dr. Eugene Narrett, a newspaper columnist, wrote (in *The Pilot* on February 2, 1996) about the problems our birth-control-addicted culture has caused in relationships between men and women:

> In a world of emergency contraception, a man, even a husband, is just a creature out there somewhere, useful for contriving a bit of excitement whose residue [a baby—Ed.] needs eradication. . . . Having fallen from assisting life to preventing it, this clinical duo [a woman and her doctor] displaces relationships based on spousal commitment and creates a new morality in which 'doctors and family planning clinics' (i.e. child prevention clinics) must face reality and give women an extra supply of birth control pills.

> Sex truly is unprotected today, endlessly exposed in public, the subject of sickening self-disclosures on television and cold-blooded analyses in mainstream papers. The mystery and joy of husband and wife and the bond between the generations decays into a messy leisure activity whose unwanted side-effects [babies—Ed.] trigger chemical interventions—on demand.

A child should not have to pay with his life for the bad judgment of his parents. The baby isn't the one who chose to get involved. Pregnancy is not a disease. It is the state of motherhood and fatherhood, and ideally, mothers and fathers should take care in the nurturing of their children.

If a woman does think she is pregnant and needs assistance, there are more than 3,500 centers around the United States with counselors and other volunteers who will help her and her baby both during the pregnancy and afterward, if necessary. The choice for life is supported in every community. Help for both mother and child is a phone call away.

Medical abortion as birth control

Today we are in the era of birth control, with drugs that will kill tiny boys and girls several weeks after their lives begin. Not only is the child going to die, but many mothers will also die—or be maimed for life.

Why do some people call these drugs birth control and not just call them abortion drugs?

Medical abortion is the correct term. No one should ever refer to these drugs as "birth control," unless one truly believes that a dead baby is always the goal of birth control.

Medical abortion is a term developed by the abortion lobby (pro-abortion groups, researchers, pharmaceutical firms and mainstream medical organizations). They believe this gives women a sense that their babies are going to die in a more private way. The promoters of these new chemicals claim that women will feel better about aborting a preborn baby if the abortion can be done earlier, without surgery and with—they say— greater privacy.

You now know that many of the chemicals women think are birth control are really deadly to tiny boys and girls. It really is not too surprising, then, that the people who have promoted birth control for so many years would continue to refine their chemical weapons so that tiny boys and girls can be killed later and later in their young lives in the womb.

The vast majority of women who use these methods of "birth control" do not realize that the chemicals can act to abort their tiny babies, but the people who have promoted the acceptance of birth control in our culture *do* know—and have always known—the truth.

MTX (Methotrexate) + Misoprostol

MTX (Methotrexate) was approved by the FDA as a cancer treatment drug. It is also used to treat psoriasis and rheumatoid arthritis, but it is an extremely toxic drug.

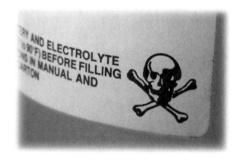

Warnings published in pharmacy reference books state: "MTX has caused fetal death and congenital anomalies . . . women of child bearing potential should not receive MTX until pregnancy is excluded and they should be fully counseled on the serious risk to the fetus should they become pregnant while undergoing treatment. . . . Do not administer to pregnant . . . patients."

MTX is so highly toxic that many who treat cancer will use this drug only as a last resort.

In the early 1980's, MTX was used to chemically destroy ectopic pregnancies. An ectopic pregnancy is one in which the baby has lodged in the mother's fallopian tube. When this occurs, both the baby *and* the mother will die if the situation is left untreated. However, when MTX was supposedly being used to treat ectopic pregnancy, the abortion-causing properties of MTX were also apparently being measured.

MTX on its own will not complete an abortion, since MTX kills the preborn baby, but leaves the child's body inside the womb.

Therefore, the mother who has an MTX medical abortion must also have a second drug, misoprostol (also known as Cytotec, used for treating ulcers).

Misoprostol is a prostaglandin, which causes contractions so that the baby will be expelled from the mother once the MTX has killed him or her. This also means that a mother who medically aborts her child using this method will make at least three visits to the abortion facility:

First visit: The woman receives an injection of MTX.

Second visit (a few days later): The woman acquires a vaginal suppository (misoprostol) which she can use at home to begin uterine contractions.

Third visit: She returns to the abortion facility for an examination to determine if the abortion is complete.

The abortion facility must also be prepared, if needed, to perform a surgical abortion on the woman should the medical abortion fail.

It is too early to know the whole truth about the many serious side effects this combination of drugs will have on women, but here is a partial listing: liver disease; negative effects on the immune system; lowering of white blood cell count (which increases the chances of infection); nausea; fever; chills; vomiting; severe cramping, and, in one case, severe bleeding that required a transfusion.

Those who use MTX are additionally warned not to take any anti-inflammatory medication or have vaccinations of any kind.[33, 34]

One of the most serious concerns is whether such chemical combinations' side effects will harm the children these women may bear later in their lives—effects that may even be passed along to their children's children. These deadly chemicals may well harm future generations of the women who have used them, but no long-term research has been done.

RU-486 + Misoprostol

RU-486 (mifepristone) is part of a chemical family known as antiprogesterones. RU-486 blocks the hormone that helps develop the lining of the uterus during pregnancy (progesterone). This lining is the source of nutrition and protection for the developing baby.

RU-486 works by starving the tiny boy or girl in the womb. It alters the lining of the uterus, thus cutting off nourishment to the tiny human being. RU-486 can accomplish this killing up to the preborn child's ninth week of life.

After RU-486 is given, the woman must return to the doctor or the clinic for a second drug, misoprostol (Cytotec). RU-486 starves the baby to death; the misoprostol causes contractions so that the baby is expelled from the womb.

In all, an RU-486 abortion may require three visits to the abortion facility, though two visits are said to be more common.

First visit: Day 1—The woman goes to the facility for a physical exam, blood test, urine test and ultrasound. Three RU-486 tablets are given to be taken orally.

At home: Day 3—The woman herself administers four tablets of misoprostol (Cytotec) by placing them in her vagina. She rests for several hours while cramping, bleeding and the actual abortion of her baby occurs.

Second visit: Day 7—The woman returns for an ultrasound to determine whether the abortion is complete. If it is not, four more misoprostol tablets are placed in her vagina.

Third visit: Day 15—The woman returns for another vaginal ultrasound. If she is still pregnant, a surgical abortion is performed.

Tragically, at least two women (one in France, one in Iowa) are known to have died from using this chemical. The other side effects include heart attack, hemorrhage, diarrhea, nausea, cramping and incomplete abortion.

An incomplete abortion means that all or part of the baby remains in the mother's uterus. At that point the woman must go in for a surgical abortion. This is why Planned Parenthood, which is testing RU-486 in several of its clinics, has announced that it will use RU-486 only in locations where an abortionist is on hand in case an incomplete abortion occurs.

Birth Control: The Legacy

"The human being in the womb has been devalued to the point of being viewed as human waste."

Birth Control: The Legacy

What are the long-term implications for our society of the latest advances in the birth control/abortion field?

In the early days of the birth control revolution in the 1960's, the Pill was called "menstrual regulation" to hide the fact that a tiny human being would be destroyed. Today, medical abortion is being heralded as one simple procedure that can be done in the privacy of one's home.

Pharmaceutical companies and abortion proponents are trumpeting this newest advance in abortion while failing to point out the hazards, the total lack of privacy and the arduous process the mother must experience before her baby dies.

The implications are mind-boggling, because it is clearly apparent that the human being who lives in the womb has been devalued to the point of being viewed as human waste.

Bioethicist Gonzalo Herranz wrote in 1985 of this latest "advance" in birth control technology:

> The significance of this type of abortion is extremely important. It will establish as an admitted social fact that the human embryo is a mere product or debris. Not only is the embryo made into a thing, stripping it of all its human value; it is reduced to the negative condition of excrement [human waste]. In the same

way that a laxative is capable of freeing a sluggish colon of its fecal contents, the new pill will enable the gestating uterus to free itself from the embryo growing within.

But perhaps the greatest tragedy is that we as a society do not seem to have learned very much. In 1937, *Physical Culture* magazine published an article titled "Will New Birth Control End Abortion Evil?" Author John Hayden wrote: "Birth control is on its way in; and once it becomes generally established, abortion will be on its way out."

Mr. Hayden could not have imagined a day when birth control would *become* abortion. But that's what has happened, and we now read about children being nothing more than "unwanted side effects."

There is something wrong with a society that sets the joy of sex above and apart from the value of a human being.

Is there any good news about birth control?

Chastity is possible. It's tough, but it's possible.

Natural methods of spacing children, known as natural family planning (NFP), have remarkable efficiency, effectiveness and a total absence of complications. The proper use of natural methods of spacing children (NFP) is analogous to ecology. Just as we strive to make sure that our rivers are clean, our air is clean and our environment is as free of toxins as possible, we should practice good body ecology. There is no reason to pollute your body with chemicals, devices, implants, or injectibles when there are natural ways to regulate fertility and plan children.

NFP is not birth control. Couples who use it realize that should their NFP result in a child, that child is a gift from God—not a "mistake." NFP is exactly what the name implies: a technique that is totally natural, easy to learn, and has wonderful, healthy side effects. It does not pollute the body, and it enriches the relationship between husband and wife.

Let's talk about the husband and wife for a moment.

Once a woman becomes familiar with her body's messages regarding her fertility, she is empowered with the ability to understand, in a most basic way, why her body was designed the way it was. She also learns how she can effectively plan, in a serious circumstance and together with her husband, to space her family.

Whereas sex outside of marriage has brought anguish and frustration to so many people and has resulted in children conceived out of wedlock, NFP promotes spousal love—sexual relations within the context of marriage—bringing forth a union of two people in spiritual, emotional and physical ways. NFP costs nothing except time and commitment.

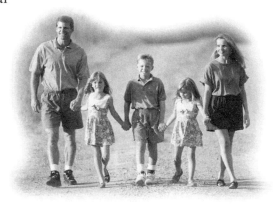

While more than 50 percent of all marriages end in divorce, it is very rare for spouses using Natural Family Planning to divorce (2 to 5 percent).[35]

Get to know more about NFP. Familiarize yourself with the easy learning techniques and make a decision based on all the facts.

It is never too late to celebrate the natural wonder of your sexuality!

So married couples should rethink their use of birth control too?

Nature is remarkable. Imagine how amazing it is for two people, who become one in marriage, to procreate another human being! This is especially thrilling when we contemplate the awesome reality of a tiny human being, no larger than the head of a pin, growing and unique in every way.

The ability to procreate is a special gift, and it should be saved for marriage. We as a society need to understand that when a man and a woman make a commitment to a lifetime of love in the real world, their commitment comes with no guarantees. There may be no picket fence around the perfect home. There may be heartache and financial reversal, but love grows stronger in times of trial. Amid these everyday realities, how could a child ever be viewed as anything other than a gift that surpasses all other gifts?

We hear in our society that children are expensive, that they are time-consuming, that they affect lifestyles in a negative way. In fact, if we were to listen to many of society's messages, we might look on the procreation of a child as a major problem. But that is not reality. It is fanatical rhetoric, bent on viewing people solely as consumers—in doubt about the value of marriage, in doubt about our own personal ability to be chaste before marriage, and in doubt about the promise of love and affection that grows in a marriage built on total self-giving and trust.

Birth control within marriage is a practice of distrust. It says the spouses cannot work together to plan their family without a device or a chemical. It says the spouses are too selfish to alter their lives for the sake of a child. And, sadly, it might say in our age of soap-opera mentality: "If you are temporarily sterile, my dear, then an affair might spice up your life!"

Birth control within marriage robs the couple of so much and is ultimately an illicit and immoral choice. Because God is the Author of life, we must trust Him—as well as each other. We must follow God's rules rather than man's rules if our love is truly destined to achieve the heights He desires us to reach.

One final thought

Perhaps this book makes you wonder whether there is something wrong with the messages our culture sends to young people. After all, if enough of the right information were made available, young people would not feel such enormous pressure to become sexually active. In fact, because young people are human beings and not animals, society is abusing them by assuming that they cannot practice self-control, by providing them with dangerous chemicals and devices with no warning, and by encouraging behaviors that are morally wrong.

We must, as human beings and children of God, be aware of the illicit practices promoted in a society that has lost its moral compass. How can we expect more from the younger generation than we have given them when we have consciously taken moral absolutes away from them?

Young people are tremendous human beings with intelligence and character. They need to be treated as human beings before we can expect, in return, that they will behave with self-respect and self-control. What will it take for us to learn such a simple lesson?

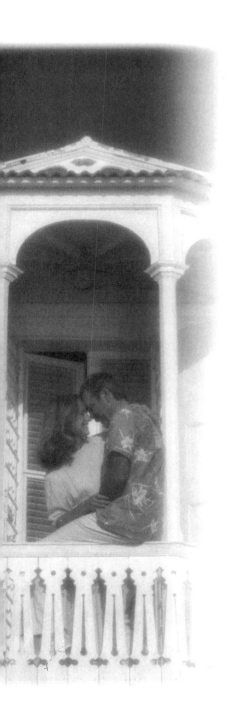

Footnotes
and
References

Footnotes

[1] Dr. Hugh K. Barber, "Statement of Editorial Purpose," *The Female Patient*, 4/96, p. 14.

[2] Lionel Tiger, "Nasty Turns in Family Life," *U.S. News and World Report*, 7/1/96, p. 57.

[3] Dr. Janet E. Smith, "The Connection Between Contraception and Abortion," One More Soul, 1996.

[4] Dr. Thomas M. Hooton, et al., "A Prospective Study of Risk Factors for Symptomatic Urinary Tract Infection in Young Women," *New England Journal of Medicine*, 8/15/96, Vol. 335, No. 7, pp. 468–474.

[5] C.D. Lytle, et al., "Filtration Sizes of Human Immunodeficiency Virus Type 1 and Surrogate Viruses Used to Test Barrier Materials," *Applied and Environmental Microbiology*, 2/92, Vol. 58, No. 2.

[6] K.D. Bird, *AIDS*, 1991, Vol. 5, pp. 791–796.

[7] B. Voeller, *AIDS*, 1992, Vol. 6, pp. 341–342. For more information, contact American Life League for our "Condoms and AIDS Fact Sheet."

[8] Stanley K. Henshaw and Jane Silverman, "The Characteristics and Prior Contraceptive Use of U. S. Abortion Patients," *Family Planning Perspectives*, 7/88, Vol. 20, No. 4, pp. 158–168.

[9] Bruce M. Carlson, *Human Embryology and Developmental Biology*, Mosby–Year Book, Inc., 1994, p. 23.

[10] Ibid., p. 31; William J. Larsen, *Human Embryology*, Churchill Livingstone, 1993, p. 13. Ronan O'Rahilly and Fabiola Muller, *Human Embryology and Teratology*, New York: Wiley-Liss, 1994, p. 19.

[11] Larsen, op. cit., p. 4.

[12] Alan E. H. Emery, *Elements of Medical Genetics*, New York: Churchill Livingstone, 1983, p. 93. Benjamin Lewin (Ed.), *Genes III*, New York: John Wiley and Sons, 1983, pp. 9–13, 20–203, and 681.

[13] Larsen, op. cit., p. 1; O'Rahilly and Muller, op. cit., p. 20.

[14] Carlson, op. cit., p. 31; Larsen, op. cit., pp. 4–5.

[15] Carlson, op. cit., p. 33.

[16] Carlson, op. cit., p. 44.

[17] Carlson, op. cit., p. 45.

[18] O'Rahilly and Muller, op. cit., p. 35.

[19] O'Rahilly and Muller, op. cit., pp. 60–63.

[20] O'Rahilly and Muller, op. cit., p. 63.

[21] "U.S. to Advance Use of the Pill," *New York Times*, 6/29/96, pp. A1, B6.

[22] John Wilks, *A Consumer's Guide to the Pill and Other Drugs*, TGB Books, 1996, p. 19.

[23] *Communiqué*, 11/1/96, p. 1.

[24] "Preferred Ignorance and the Bitter Pill," *The National Reporter*, 9–10/96, p. 3.

[25] Ibid.

[26] Irving Sivin, "IUDs Are Contraceptives, Not Abortifacients: A Comment on Research and Belief," *Studies in Family Planning*, 12/89, Vol. 20, No. 6, pp. 355–359.

[27] Editorial comment on "Patient Satisfaction and Side Effects With Levonorgestrel Implant (Norplant) Use in Adolescents 18 Years of Age or Younger," *Obstetrics and Gynecological Survey*, 4/94, p. 272.

[28] Wilks, op. cit., pp. 81–88.

[29] "Answers to the Catholic Physicians' Guild Quiz," *Newsletter of the Catholic Physicians' Guild*, 7/95.

[30] "Fears Keeping 'After Sex' Pill on Back Shelf," *Chicago Tribune*, 2/14/96, pp. 1, 8.

[31] Wilks, op. cit., p. 133.

[32] Ann Landers, "'Morning-After' Tablets Aren't Always Effective," *Free Lance-Star*, 5/19/87.

[33] Dr. Ellen Wiebe, "Abortion Induced With Methotrexate and Misoprostol," *Canadian Medical Association Journal*, 1/15/96, Vol. 154, No. 2, pp. 165–170.

[34] Methotrexate complete description, America Online, from *Consumer Reports Complete Drug Reference*.

[35] Mercedes Arzu Wilson, *Love and Family*, Ignatius Press, 1996, p. 261.

References for Further Reading:

The following items are available from American Life League:

The *Life Guide* series:

> *The Facts of Life*
> *The Facts About Birth Control*
> *The Facts About Abortion*
> *Title X: The Six-Billion Dollar Scam*
> *Reflections on Suffering*
> *What About Self-Esteem?*
> *Tips When You're Pregnant and Need Help*
> *The Facts About Post-Abortion Syndrome*
> *The Facts About Mercy Killing*
> *The Culture of Death*
> *Living Life Principles*
> *The Reproductive Technology Lie*

A Consumer's Guide to the Pill and Other Drugs by John Wilks

Pope Paul VI, Modern Day Prophet by William F. Colliton, Jr., M.D.

Contraception and Evangelium Vitae

Infant Homicides through Contraceptives by Bogomir Kuhar

Other references:

The Doctor's Case against the Pill by Barbara Seaman, Hunter House, 1995.

Humanae Vitae: A Generation Later by Dr. Janet E. Smith, The Catholic University of America Press, 1991.

Why Humanae Vitae Was Right: A Reader edited by Dr. Janet E. Smith, Ignatius Press, 1993.

To obtain further assistance, please contact:

One More Soul
616 Five Oaks Ave.
Dayton, OH 45406
(800) 307-7685

Pastors for Life
229 Siloam Rd.
Easley, SC 29642
(864) 220-6317

Pharmacists for Life International
P.O. Box 1281
Powell, OH
(800) 227-8359
e-mail: pfli@ix.netcom.com
web: http://www.netcom.com/~pfli/cc.html

Protestants Against Birth Control
P.O. Box 07240
Milwaukee, WI 53207
(414) 483-3399

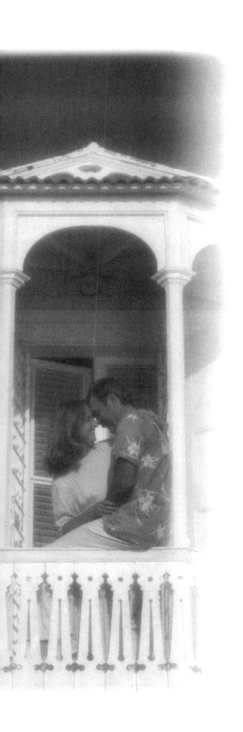

Appendix

Appendix:

Society's Love Affair with Death: A Commentary on the Contraceptive Mentality

by Father Denis O'Brien, M.M.,
Spiritual Director, American Life League, Inc.

What is a contraceptive mentality?

Increasingly, those intrepid souls who persevere in the struggle to defend the dignity of human life ask themselves why more attention is not paid to the connection between contraception and abortion. Apparently, some pro-life leaders look upon contraception as not so bad, or, if it is bad or maybe somewhat immoral, as something that should be tolerated passively as a lesser evil in order to obtain a greater good—namely, a decrease in the number of abortions on demand. Leaving aside the fact that many oral contraceptives are not contraceptives at all but really abortifacients and that others may have a high failure rate or possibly produce teratogenic (abnormal development) effects on the preborn child, where did the idea originate that one may do evil in order to obtain a good?

It is one thing to have to put up with a lesser evil in order to avoid a greater evil or to promote a greater good, but it is never permissible to do evil so that good may be brought about. Using a contraceptive is a voluntary act of doing what is intrinsically evil.

After World War II, the Nuremberg trials made clear that society will hold each person responsible for his or her actions. Claiming that "I only obeyed orders" was not accepted as a valid excuse for such crimes as torturing prisoners. In the same way, no one may claim that "I was forced to resort to contraception" in order to keep the family from increasing.

If pro-life speakers so much as mention the word "contraception" during a conference they can sense a certain coolness come into the minds of a good number of their listeners. Just the same, we will never destroy the acceptance of procured abortion from the field of human activity until we learn that contraception is the root of abortion. We have to uproot the contraceptive mentality because it breeds an anti-life mentality, although contraceptive users may sincerely believe that they are pro-life.

Some seem to think that treating the problem of contraceptive converts the issue of life from a human issue into a conservative Catholic issue. Yet it is the mentality that will affect the "to be or not to be" of millions of human beings. If one believes that having babies *only* when one wants them (as if man and wife themselves were empowered to say, "Let there be life!") and that spacing children by means of the pill are OK, then one must accept the notion that if an unplanned pregnancy should somehow occur, and the baby is not wanted, the parents may, in effect, stop talking about their *baby* and begin to plan how to dispose of *it* by means of an OK abortion. The "slippery slope" is named Mount Contraceptive.

Efforts to promote the dignity of human life will never be understood or make any sense outside of the context that God is alive and well and is still the only Author of life, still the only One allowed to decide not only who shall live and who must die today, but whether a life should be conceived or not. The right to life includes God's right to give life.

When we speak of God we are referring to the Almighty, without beginning or end, who offers us a kingdom and proposes a change of heart to obtain it, who has revealed Himself as our Father. Thus abortion is the murder of an innocent brother or sister. None of us could ask for life. We did not exist. Life is a gift from God, a boon that makes us in His image and His likeness endowing us with a dignity little less than angelic. We are partly spirit. We can reason and remember and laugh and plan. Our disappointments do not depend on a Pavlovian reflex. We are also matter—very important matter since the Word became flesh, was born of a woman and dwelt among us, died, rose, and ascended into heaven for us.

When God made each one of us unique, He gave us the power to enter into a uniquely intimate relation with one of the opposite sex. He blesses this union for the validly married and even crowns it with another power—that of collaborating with Him in the transmission of new life, when He so wills. To use any contraceptive is to say to God that this permanent good, not a mere utility for a happy hour in matrimony, is in reality an evil, an impediment to living precisely as one wants.

We are always bound to obey God. The moral law binds always or it never binds. It binds totally or it does not bind it all. Actions follow beliefs. The contraceptive mentality is sex without responsibility. Union dedicated to sterility. Fun and games—never grow up. Sex machine. No worries. But this is precisely what Satan so cunningly assured Eve: Not to worry. You won't die. You'll be like gods. But Adam and Eve did die, and they didn't become like gods. Nobody tells God how to set the rules for life. If men and women want to marry they have the right to do so (other things being equal). But God has set the rules, according to which this life is the antechamber to the next.

"God is not mocked," St. Paul tells us, and this is the first reason why the contraceptive mentality is linked to abortion (and now to euthanasia, genetic manipulation, fetal experimentation and *in vitro* fertilization): Men may not pick and choose when it comes to morality. God is like a technician who wires a computer. All is perfect. But if the operator does not operate the machine correctly he will get "garbage in, garbage out." Men have to check the manual of the Ten Commandments constantly before they operate the computer of life. Man is still clay; he may not give orders to the Potter. Man may not tell God how the norms for the transmission of life are to be established.

Contraception breeds abortion

More than one writer has pointed out the connection.

A. "The current belief that illegitimacy will be reduced if teenage girls are given an effective contraceptive is an extension of the same reasoning that created the problem in the first place. It reflects the willingness to face problems of social control and discipline while trusting some technical device to extricate society from its difficulties. The irony is that our current rise in illegitimacy has occurred precisely while contraception was becoming more rather than less widespread and respectable" (Dr. Kingsley Davis, *The American Family in Relation to Demographic Change*).

B. "Better techniques for early abortion have also proved to be an important backup in human clinical trials of new drugs and devices where contraceptive efficacy is not fully determined. Increasingly, investigators are under pressure to establish the minimal effective dose for contraceptive drugs but medical ethics require that the human subjects in such tests be protected from unwanted pregnancy by access to safe abortion. . . .

"In the not-too-distant future, it may be possible for a woman to bring on a missed menstrual period by simply inserting a vaginal suppository, taking an injection, or swallowing a pill." (Theodore M. King, M.D., "Abortion and Abortifacients," *Draper Fund Report*, No. 6, Summer, 1978, pp. 27–30).

C. "Margaret Sanger, the foundress of Planned Parenthood in the United States, had condoned abortion in her 1916 edition of *Family Limitation*, stating that 'No one can doubt that abortion is justifiable.' But her colleague Havelock Ellis helped persuade her to change her public stance on the matter, shrewdly advising her that the 'right to create or not create new life' had better propaganda value than the 'right to destroy.' As a result, Margaret Sanger began using abortion as a lever to make contraception more acceptable, arguing that contraception would put an end to abortion. Abortions are 'barbaric,' she than exclaimed, and classified it with infanticide as 'the killing of babies.'" (Dr. Donald DeMarco, *The Contraceptive Mentality and Abortion*, 1982, p. 5).

D. "The grim reality of the situation is seen by the doctor in his consulting rooms. Into them comes a constant stream of girls and parents, full of tears, often pregnant, sometimes with veneral infections, living in sordid circumstances, the beauty and innocence of childhood long since lost. The parents utter what has now become the standard *cri de coeur* 'Where have we gone wrong?' In fact they have not gone wrong anywhere. There is a war on and the children are the casualties. They were promised by the glossy magazines and the silver screen a good time and happiness in sex, and all they finish up with is suffering and disillusionment. Love dies and leaves only broken hearts.

This should cause us no surprise. Almost a century ago Sigmund Freud said that sexual abnormality leads on to sadism and masochism. He was referring to the more exotic forms of sexual activity but the same principle holds for extramarital intercourse. In the thirteenth century St. Thomas Aquinas, whose intellect and insight were exceeded only by his sanctity, said: 'Impurity leads inevitably to violence.'" (H.P. Dunn, Kt.St. S., FRCS, FRCOG, FRACS, *Sex and Sensibility*, 1983, p. 19).

Contraception becomes abortion

Recently, Robert G. Marshall and Charles A. Donovan co-authored a blockbuster about contraception: *Blessed Are the Barren* (San Francisco: *Ignatius Press*, 1991). The remarkably well-documented study shines a very bright light into some very dark corners. For example:

During a 1955 conference on abortion, Dr. Kinsey himself said:

At the risk of being repetitious, I would remind the group that we have found the highest frequency of induced abortion in the group which, in general, most frequently used contraceptives.

Dr. Christopher Tietze has made it known that:

a high correlation between abortion experience and contraceptive experience can be expected in populations to which both contraception and abortion are available and where some couples have attempted to regulate the number and spacing of their children.

Let us not forget the Third World:

Mariano Requena has found that in Latin America the introduction of more effective contraception led to an increase in the abortion rate.

Dr. Bernard Nathanson reviewed *The Abortion Pill: RU-486* by Etienne-Emile Baulieu (New York: Simon & Schuster) in *National Review*, February 3, 1992, pp. 47–48. Dr. Nathanson was one of the founders of the National Abortion Rights Action League in 1969. He says in his review that he has done or directed more than 75,000 abortions. He compares the trial for RU-486 to the Willowbrook experiments in which live hepatitis virus was injected into mentally retarded children at the Willowbrook Institution on Staten Island. The families of the children were assured that "the live virus was good for them." Baulieu, the self-styled designer of the abortion pill, rejects any comparison with the DES experience, in which pregnant women were supposed to be protected from a threatened miscarriage and would also help pregnant women who suffered from diabetes. A significant number of those women's daughters were seen some ten to fifteen years later to be suffering from a ferocious variant of cancer of the vagina. RU-486 has no long period of testing for safety. Like DES, RU-486 is a synthetic female hormone.

Baulieu says that the word "abortion" is too traumatic (he must, then, be unable to express the horror of the deed), so he wants to call RU-486 "contragestive" instead of "abortifacient." Galveston Right to Life puts this effort in its proper perspective: "This is equivalent to classifying a guillotine as a 'headache prevention device'" (*RU-486— The Death Pill*).

Baulieu himself admits (after trying to refute Raymond J. Godfroid's warnings about the safety of his product) that:

Finally, Mr. Godfroid is correct in saying that pregnancy termination is a "traumatic event." It is indeed all the more traumatizing for the often irrational, emotionally charged debate that surrounds it. I proposed the term 'contragestion' not in any way so as to hide the real function of the drug, but rather to avoid the systematic mind blocks that are created by charged terminology [Letter to *The Journal of the American Medical Association*, February 16, 1990, p. 948].

Well, if a rose by any other name smells just as sweet, abortion by any other name still smells of murder.

Professor Jerome Lejeune, who was almost certainly the world's most distinguished geneticist, succinctly disposes of the term "contragestive." He calls RU-486 the "human pesticide." It is a chemical product that prevents or interrupts the fertilized egg from implanting in the uterus.

Those who continue to insist that contraception and abortion are two completely distinct problems may be interested in reading what transpired in the U.S. Supreme Court on April 26, 1989. In his oral argument in the case of *Webster v. Reproductive Health Services*, Frank Susman, representing Reproductive Health Services, stated that the rights to contracept and to abort "because of advances in medicine and science, now overlap. They coalesce and merge and they are not distinct." Justice Scalia did not see why there was not a separation between contraception and abortion. Mr. Susman replied:

If I may suggest the response in your question, Justice Scalia. The most common forms of what we generically in common parlance call contraception today—IUDs, low-dose birth control pills, which are the safest type of birth control pills available—act as abortifacients. They are correctly labeled as such.

Under this statute, which defines fertilization as the point of beginning, those forms of contraception are also abortifacients. Science and medicine refers to them as both. We are not still dealing with the common barrier methods of Griswold. We are no longer just talking about condoms and diaphragms. Things have changed. The bright line, if there ever was one, has now been extinguished. That's why I suggest to this court that we need to deal with one right, the right to procreate. We are no longer talking about two rights [*Washington Post*, April 27, 1989, p. A16].

Catholic thought and the contraceptive mentality

Later Catholic authors treat directly of contraception and abortion in the same moral context. Tertullian, for example, wrote in the *Apologia* (9.8) that "He destroys a man who destroys a man-to-be." Minucius Felix in *Octavius*, the early third century *Elenchos* (9.12.5), St. Ambrose, Bishop of Milan, in *Hexaemeron* (5.18.58), St. Jerome, in letter 22, *To Eustochium* (13), St. Caesarius of Arles, in Sermons 1,12, the *Irish Collection of Canons* ("Womanly Questions" 3.3) and the St. Hubert Penitential (ch. 56) teach the same.

Si aliquis, an ancient canon of uncertain origin, which declared that an attempt to prevent generation or cause sterility was to be considered homicide, was part of Church legislation from 1232 to 1917. Pope Gregory IX ordered Raymond of Penafort to compile the canons and decrees of his predecessors. The first universal legislation by a Pope against contraception, contained in the *Decretals of Gregory* IX (4.5.7) contained *Si conditiones*; it declared null any marriage entered into with a condition of avoiding children. For more detailed information, the reader is invited to consult *The New Catholic Encyclopedia* in order to read "Contraception" and "Decretals of Gregory IX."

The Roman Catechism published in 1565 a synthesis of the teaching and ecclesiastical discipline that was agreed to and voted on at Trent, then approved by the Pope. Pope St. Pius V instructed that it be published. A part of the teaching on marriage simply repeats what the Church, always protected from error by Jesus Christ, has taught from the beginning, because the apostles were instructed to go and teach all nations to obey everything He had commanded them. The Council Fathers at Trent were bound to hold fast to the deposit of faith; they could not change what Christ had taught, nor could they pretend to "invent" new teachings. And this is what they said:

> A second reason for marriage is the desire of family, not so much, however, with a view to leave after us heirs to inherit our property and fortune, as to bring up children in the true faith and in the service of God. That such was the principal object of the holy Patriarchs when they married is clear from Scripture. Hence the Angel, when informing Tobias of the means of repelling the violent assaults of the evil demon, says: *I will show thee who they are over whom the devil can prevail; for they who in such manner receive matrimony as to shut out God from themselves and from their mind, and to give themselves to their lust, as the horse and mule which have not understanding, over them the devil hath power. He then adds: Thou shalt take the virgin with the fear of the Lord, moved rather for love of children than for lust, that in the seed of Abraham thou mayest obtain a blessing in children.* It was also for this reason that God instituted marriage from the beginning; and therefore married persons who, to prevent conception or procure abortion, have recourse to medicine, are guilty of a most heinous crime—nothing less than wicked conspiracy to commit murder. [*Roman Catechism, Part 2, The Sacraments* (Rockford, IL: Tan Books, 1982, p. 344)].

Good Pope John XXIII's wish to open a few windows has often, too often, been interpreted as a desire to "get with" the modern world. Actually, he wanted the post-World War II world to "get with" the Gospel, as he made clear in his opening address to the Bishops at the Second Vatican Council. And it was precisely in the pastoral document "The Church in the Modern World," which the Fathers composed and Paul VI approved, in the long section on marriage and the family, that:

> in questions of birth regulation the sons of the Church, faithful to these principles, are forbidden to use methods disapproved by the teaching authority of the Church in its interpretation of the divine law [No. 51].

How could the Church change what Christ taught? Christ is the same yesterday, today and forever. He is the Head and we are the body of the Church. If we call ourselves followers of Christ, may we take out His teaching and put in our fallible judgments?

Caveat emptor: Let the buyer beware!

What Susman referred to as advances in medicine and science appeal to many people. Still, there are other experts, just as learned and equally qualified in the fields of medicine and science who look beyond pragmatism and the bottom line to long-range effects. One of those was Dr. William Lynch, who taught Ob-Gyn at Tufts Medical College. He never wearied of reminding not only his students and his patients but anyone else who would listen to him that "it takes ten years to know what a new discovery will do for you and it takes twenty years to find out what it will do to you."

All the advances, if one insists upon calling them that, do not subtract one jot or tittle from the import of Pope John Paul II's teaching. Whether by means of a drug or by means of a pill or by hacking body parts asunder or by suction, or by using an IUD, whether the victim is eight days old or eight weeks old or eight months old, the cold and deliberate destruction of that innocent person is still murder—in the true and proper sense of the word. Call it a fetus if you will. Just don't forget that "fetus" is the Latin word for baby.

Isn't it interesting that when people do not want to have a *baby* they try to prevent *conception*? But if pregnancy does occur, and a *baby* is still not desired, the people involved use the la-la land rationalization to simply "terminate the pregnancy" (just what was the woman carrying?) and dispose of the "product of conception." Could we have some details about the product? If a person is not aborted, how shall we explain post-abortion syndrome? In the case of a botched abortion, why do some women say with regret, "I killed the only child I will ever have"?

Contraception is not perhaps wrong at times because it breaches some ecclesiastical code or some sectarian consensus; it is always intrinsically evil because it violates the eternal law of God, the only Author of matrimony just as He is the only Author of life.

The determination to defend the right to life and the respect for life on behalf of everyone must be founded on that divine law and act in accordance with it. If the issue of contraception divides the respect-life effort, regrettably, divided we stand, though the heavens fall.

This material is excerpted from an original booklet entitled *The Piller of Society*, first published by American Life League in 1981. Copious updates could have been added, but history does not need to be updated, it needs to be learned. Those who refuse to learn are doomed to repeat the mistakes of the past; and in this case, that means that human beings will die if the lesson is not learned and heeded.

The author of this material, Father Denis O'Brien, M.M. has been the spiritual director of American Life League since its founding in 1979. We are grateful to him for guiding us ever on the path to Truth: no diverison, no excuses.

He has taught us well: Always speak the truth and let the chips fall where they may.

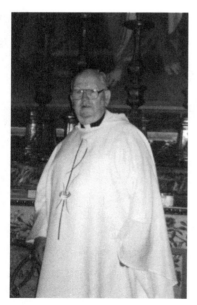

Photo of Father Denis O'Brien celebrting his 44th anniversary as a Maryknoll priest by saying Mass at St. Peter's Basilica, Vatican City, June 13, 1997.

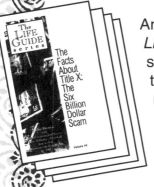